THE STATE PROVISION OF SANATORIUMS

THE STATE PROVISION
OF SANATORIUMS

BY

S. V. PEARSON,

M.D. (Cantab.), M.R.C.P. (London)

Cambridge:

at the University Press

1913

CAMBRIDGE UNIVERSITY PRESS
Cambridge, New York, Melbourne, Madrid, Cape Town,
Singapore, São Paulo, Delhi, Tokyo, Mexico City

Cambridge University Press
The Edinburgh Building, Cambridge CB2 8RU, UK

Published in the United States of America by Cambridge University Press, New York

www.cambridge.org
Information on this title: www.cambridge.org/9780521232982

First published 1913
First paperback edition 2011

A catalogue record for this publication is available from the British Library

ISBN 978-0-521-23298-2 Paperback

PREFACE

THE subject of public health is one of perennial interest, but it is one which has come especially to the fore lately. The sanatorium treatment of consumption was advocated as long ago as 1840 by Bodington; in recent years it has come into vogue to a wide extent; but even now it is ill-understood and not always accepted. The advent of the National Insurance Act has brought the subject of the State provision of sanatoriums acutely forward, and has aroused a widespread interest not only in the medical, but also in the economic aspects of the subject.

I have for some years been keenly interested in the many-sided influence of sanatoriums. I have attempted in the following pages to deal from a practical point of view with the complicated questions involved in the State provision of these institutions. At the same time I have tried to reach some of the guiding principles underlying the various problems involved, principles often difficult to arrive at and to grasp. There is still too little coordination between the authorities responsible for the provision of sana-toriums, and too weak a driving force behind them.

But the apparent chaos which strikes bewilderment into the minds of many unacquainted with the details of the fight against tuberculosis will be dispelled by the acquisition of fuller knowledge. Much is still only just being begun. Many things are in a transition stage. Nevertheless I feel a useful purpose can be served by gathering together here a few facts and opinions culled by one who for nearly a decade has been in the thick of the fight.

Some fear too much zeal. Recently a delegate to a conference in Paris said, the problem of the future would be how the healthy ten per cent. of the population could maintain the remaining ninety per cent. in institutions! But the provision of sanatoriums will not only show the advantages of the institutional treatment of the sick, it will also help to spread the gospel of hygiene, thus preventing disease; and in my estimation it will, as the direct result of eradicating tuberculosis, banish not less than one quarter of the illness now rife.

Time may alter some of my opinions, other arrangements may soon be found better than those outlined in this little book. Nevertheless it is with the hope that its perusal may prove interesting and helpful to a wide circle of readers that I publish it. I commend a study of these pages especially to that numerous band of interested and disinterested workers amongst County Councillors, doctors, and National

Health Insurance Committeemen, in whose hands the management of State sanatoriums lies. I would fain have gone more fully and deeply into many of the issues raised. I could have wished for more time to consider several points, and to amend the presentation of my views more carefully. But in many quarters the consideration of the matters I deal with are urgently pressing, and the exigencies of my every-day duties preclude me from devoting any more time at present to the subject. I pray therefore for lenience for my shortcomings and omissions.

S. VERE PEARSON.

July 1913.

LIST OF CONTENTS

CHAPTER I

INTRODUCTION

MEDICAL subjects are now recognised as social problems. Preventable disease will never be eradicated unless the social condition of the people is improved. A great impetus has been given to the crusade against conditions producing sickness by national health insurance legislation. The State provision of sanatoriums will help forward this crusade, and incidentally will counteract other social evils. For the influence of sanatoriums has always been great in teaching people the simple laws of hygiene, and the dependence of these upon common-sense and upon a correct mode of life necessitating good environmental conditions. Questions of vast importance, therefore, are : How will the State provision of sanatoriums help the crusade? And what principles can be laid down to guide people in the proper methods by which State sanatoriums are to be provided and maintained?

Before attempting to answer these two questions some explanation of what I mean by a "sanatorium," by "sanatorium treatment," and by "the State provision," is called for. By the word "sanatorium" I mean an institution in the country for the treatment of resident patients suffering from tuberculosis in any of its forms.   This definition excludes such institutions as Farm colonies.   Anyone to whom the term "patient" is applicable should not be put to work on a farm.   It is a mistake to mix up the treatment of disease with productive industry, or with such a problem as that of getting people "back to the land," a problem only quite indirectly connected with the treatment of the sick.   This is not to say that it is unwise to employ, when it can be conveniently arranged, ex-patients suitable in character and bodily fitness to work regularly about a sanatorium.   A few such afford encouragement to the other inmates, and often help considerably in the discipline and moral tone of the place, besides enabling themselves to test their capabilities and regain confidence in the reality of their recoveries.

Though my definition excludes dispensaries, I shall deal briefly with these, and with the place of the sanatorium amongst the other less important forces ranged up to combat tuberculosis.

Next, as to the meaning of sanatorium treatment, I consider the two essential features of sanatorium treatment are : firstly, the close and skilled supervision of whatever remedial measures may be advisable, whether these be the all important regulation of rest and exercise, or the administration of vaccines; secondly, the proper training of the individual in hygienic living, particularly in respect of breathing fresh air, feeding rationally, and preventing infection.   It often includes, too, the removal of the patient from the manifold deleterious influences and conditions of his home which are common.   Sanatoriums will gradually become more universally supported by members of the medical profession when doctors more fully comprehend, firstly what sanatorium treatment is, and secondly its advantages, and as the unconscious effect of being paid chiefly by the sick is by degrees superseded by a system giving doctors a more direct and universal financial interest in the curing of the patient and in the maintenance of health. Hitherto sanatorium treatment has been measured too much from the standpoint of the cure of the individual; it is the most essential method to employ for this object, but its influence is of equally great importance in the direction of education and prevention.

By the term "the State provision" I mean the provision of an institution by communal action. I shall treat the subject of "The State provision of Sanatoriums" under the following heads :

I. Remarks upon the reasons why it seems well for the State to provide and maintain such institutions, and upon the principles to follow in raising a communal fund for this purpose (Chap. ii).

II. Outline of what is being done in this and some other countries at present (Chap. iii).

III. On the methods of financing and of controlling the efficiency of State sanatoriums (Chap. iv).

IV. On other agencies for combating tuberculosis and their connection with the sanatorium (Chap. v).

CHAPTER II

WHY A STATE SHOULD PROVIDE SANATORIUMS, AND THE PRINCIPLES TO FOLLOW IN RAISING A FUND

ONCE upon a time the prevention of disease was alone considered to be the duty of the State in the sphere of public health. That view has long since been abandoned. Prevention and cure are not separable, but react indirectly upon one another. Sickness produces an economic waste which affects all. Destitution is a canker which saps the foundations of wealth. Discontent upsets the peace of the community. Sickness is the greatest propagator of destitution and discontent. Hence the necessity for all to contribute towards the eradication of disease, and towards the treatment of ill-health wherever occurring. But if all must contribute, how are the contributions to be apportioned? Most parties in a modern state agree that the wealthy must contribute a proportionately large share, but the grounds upon which the justice of this plan is based are not always thought out or agreed upon. And there is seldom any consensus of opinion as to what constitutes the best method for achieving this end. Whatever method be adopted, it must be examined critically to see whether or not the well-to-do are really paying, or whether the scheme enables them to pass on their duties to their less fortunate brethren. Again, if the communal fund for fighting disease is partly raised by contributions from insured workpeople, it must be borne in mind that these insured persons, as members of the general community, whether ratepayers or not, will themselves probably be paying directly or indirectly no small part of the money found by the local authority, or by the national exchequer.

If wealth were more equally distributed, the fair apportionment of everyone's contribution towards such institutions as sanatoriums would be rendered easier than it is at present. Some socialists believe in the possibility of an equal distribution of wealth. But the forces of nature show abhorrence of parity; and one of the ways in which human beings show their inherent connection with natural forces is by exhibiting inequality in their capabilities and in their requirements. It seems irrational therefore to suggest equality in the distribution of wealth. Rational reforms aim only at its more equal distribution.

The State does not take money from A in order to cure the ailments of B, A being rich and B poor. It gets A to contribute largely to the cure of B's ailments not so much because he is better able to pay, but because the State renders A more services than it does to B, in that it enables him to get and keep more wealth than B has. The vast riches which the few have in comparison with the many are not, as their possessors are all too wont to believe, usually or chiefly the rewards of superior intelligence, ability and industry.

These riches are to a large extent the result of the superior State services rendered to their owners. The direct rendering of these services is obscured, because political power and law-making have been, for so many generations, chiefly exercised by the owners of such wealth. They fail to appreciate properly how great an effect upon their financial status present systems of levying rates and taxes have, and how greatly land monopoly contributes directly or indirectly to their position.

Contributions from other elements of society besides the wealthy are now-a-days usually levied from employers and employed workers. When the State provides sanatoriums for the treatment of consumptive workers it calls for contributions from employers of labour, whether well-to-do or not, since expediency and justice demand that the employer should help in securing the efficiency of his human machinery, if one may so term the employees.

When the money has been raised the State does not devote it solely or even primarily to benefit the worker, but it devotes it to improve the safety, to advance the efficiency and the general level of comfort and happiness of the whole society of which both the workers and the wealthy are members. This result is achieved not only directly by the restoration to health of the worker, or by the amelioration of his condition ; but also indirectly by the educational influence, upon himself and others connected with him, of his period of treatment. Prevention and cure thus become inseparably fused together and have a reciprocating, good influence upon society. The State provision of sanatoriums may do much to teach one and all that a progressive State does not confer special advantages or favours upon one class at the expense of another, and that prevention and cure cannot be divorced.

Tuberculosis is now recognised in most civilised lands as a peculiarly important cause of sickness. Lister and Garland in their "Sanatoria for the People" count the cost of consumption to this nation as equivalent to at least twelve million pounds sterling per annum. In most lands tuberculosis is treated separately when any scheme of sickness benefit or State insurance against sickness comes to be considered. The reason of this is obvious when its chronic nature and consequent strain upon any funds created for sickness benefit are considered.

CHAPTER III

In the United Kingdom the Government provided
£1,500,000 in its Finance Act 1911, to go towards
the building of sanatoriums. This fund is to be
granted to Local Authorities, who must find a further
sum equal to ⅖ths of the total cost. Under the National
Insurance Act 1911, the sum of 1s. 3d. per insured
person was found for sanatorium treatment, and an
additional 1d. which may be utilised for research. But
of these amounts, in themselves little enough for town
dwellers, it is now arranged that 6d. per insured person
is to be utilised for the payment of domiciliary treatment by general practitioners.

Besides these funds there are various voluntary
charities for the treatment of consumption, and a few
for the treatment of other forms of tuberculosis; and
some local authorities provide considerable amounts
for the treatment of consumption, apart from the
expenditure under the Poor Law, in whose infirmaries
many indigent consumptives, generally in an advanced
stage, find residence.

The Government also arranged for a maintenance
grant from the Exchequer equal in amount to half the

cost of caring for the non-insured tuberculous patient, provided that the local authority finds the other half. Hence, matters will work out thus : local authorities which provide institutional treatment for tuberculous cases will secure repayment of their expenses from the Insurance funds in respect of insured persons to the extent that the available funds permit. After the sum repaid from the Insurance funds has been deducted all the remaining expenditure will be payable half from local rates and half from the Government contribution. It is proposed, however, that the contributions from the National Insurance funds should, at all events eventually, include payments in respect of dependants of insured persons. By these means by far the largest proportion of the total cost of treating the tuberculous comprehensively is provided out of Insurance funds or the national exchequer. This is a great advance upon previous arrangements, which placed most of the cost upon the ratepayer, and through one cause or another led to the work being incompletely and inefficiently done. It was especially deficient in that it failed to bring cases under treatment early.

It is to the advantage of the community to have all medical practitioners financially interested in getting Phthisis diagnosed early and treated adequately in a sanatorium. The authors of the Insurance Bill obviously kept this point in view. Although a strong effort was at one time made by our British Medical Association to get vast sums of money paid to general practitioners for domiciliary treatment of consumptives on the basis of a fixed tariff, the Government strove to retain for institutional treatment the bulk of the money provided for the "sanatorium benefit" of the insured. And this effort on the part of the Association was supported strenuously, and over a long period, in spite of the fact that much more adequate remuneration was being offered to doctors as tuberculosis experts than had up to then been usual. It is a sad reflection for a doctor, that the Government were decidedly in advance of the medical profession in this particular, and that the Government much more than the profession showed appreciation of the advantages of having a fixed policy both to encourage the separation of the functions of physician and pharmacist, and to discourage the abuse of drugs.

In Germany the crusade against consumption derived its main impetus from the Insurance Laws. There the bulk of the provision and maintenance of sanatoriums for the workers is undertaken by the Invalidity Insurance authorities who come under a separate organisation and separate laws from those dealing with ordinary sickness. But both the sickness insurance systems, organised on a local basis according to trades and occupations, and to a less extent the municipal bodies participate in the maintenance of sanatoriums. The cost of treatment in public institutions for the tuberculous is approximately 4*s.* 7*d.* per patient per diem (32*s.* 1*d.* a week). The Pension Boards who administer the funds of the Invalidity Insurance authorities spent £1,347,000 on curative treatment of all kinds in 1910. This treatment was almost entirely that of tuberculous patients. After deduction of all refunds (amounting to nearly £300,000) the cost to the Pension Boards themselves works out as equal to 1*s.* 4½*d.* a head per annum for all persons insured against invalidity. There must be added to this expenditure that of some of the large sickness funds which do similar work themselves, instead of contributing towards the expenses of the Pension Boards ; and in several large towns the amounts expended by the local authority, and to a much smaller extent by local voluntary charities.

All sickness funds are autonomous, subject to supervision by the communal or the State administrative authorities. As a rule a fund is governed by an executive elected by the insured persons and the employers in the proportions in which they bear the cost of contributions. But the Invalidity Insurance system is administered by independent authorities, wholly different in constitution from those administering the sickness funds, and separate contributions are levied from workpeople and employers in respect of each system.

Tuberculous patients, beneficiaries under the insurance schemes, if unattached persons, *i.e.* without dependants, can be compelled to undergo institutional treatment. Otherwise compulsory powers are for the most part absent, and are apparently not seriously required, because in Germany unwillingness to go to an institution seems to be much less prevalent than is the case in England. A partial exception to this, however, is in respect of the advanced consumptives, for the effort to segregate them has not met with complete success. The advantage of treating the sick in institutions rather than in their own homes is becoming increasingly appreciated in Germany, in spite of the fact that the immediate cost to sickness funds is higher. This is no doubt due to "the increasing recognition by the working classes of the importance of health and their willingness to make large sacrifices on its behalf[1]." It also, no doubt, depends upon docility and submissiveness to the ordering of their lives which long years of conscription, and German methods of nation-making, have inculcated.

In combating tuberculosis in Germany the establishing of dispensaries and the efforts accomplished to improve the housing of the working classes remain to be mentioned. Both these undertakings are for the most part carried out by the local authority; but the Pension Boards help better housing by advancing money at a low rate of interest. No less than £18,000,000 has been so lent. And dispensaries and clinics derive a certain amount of support, as well as supervision, from the German Central Committee, whose means are derived from subscriptions, donations, and an Imperial subsidy. In addition to these enterprises a gradually increasing number of local authorities spend money on forest resorts for adults and forest schools for children, holiday colonies, "after-care," and grants towards rent, food (particularly milk), beds and bedding. The dispensary when existing is the co-ordinating centre, and works hand in hand with other allied departments; and the general practitioners of the town and district usually co-operate cordially with it.

The distinction between insured workers and their

[1] Government paper (Cd. 6581 (1913) p. 16) on *Medical Benefit in Germany*.

dependants in respect of the receipt of benefits is variable and not well defined in Germany.   Under permissive powers many dependants of insured workers become beneficiaries.   By next year probably more than a third of the entire population of Germany will be directly affected as beneficiaries under the Insurance Laws.

By the above brief account of what is being done in Germany indications are given as to how the work of combating tuberculosis is made a national scheme, to a large extent connected with and dependent upon the insurance funds.

It is worth noting in connection with German State medicine that much trouble has arisen there through the doctors not having a pecuniary interest in keeping down the drug bill.

In Norway by the dying out of leprosy large sums have been set free.   These help to form a central fund for combating tuberculosis ; the rest of which is made up by the National Society for the Prevention of Tuberculosis.   The National Society gets funds by contributions and by the sale of the may flower.   The may flower is a little red flower sold for 10 *ore* ($1\frac{1}{2}d$.) which costs 2 *ore* to make.   It is sold by flower girls on the 1st of May.   The national movement is such a keen one that large sums are made by means of the sale of this flower.   The local rates hardly contribute at all to this central fund, nor do imperial taxes.   In the sanatoriums the poor people are subsidised, and they also pay a shilling a week for themselves ; even a respectable artisan, however, does not contribute more than about 1*s*. 6*d*. a week.   With respect to the medical profession, there are whole-time sanatorium doctors, but there are no whole-time dispensary doctors. The municipal nursing homes exist solely for tuberculosis. The doctors of these are general practitioners. These homes are sorting-houses, and diagnosis houses; originally they were for hopeless cases, now they are for all. It was found that they were too unpopular to gain support when they were confined to the reception of hopeless cases. Doctors are encouraged to learn sanatorium methods. Norway is divided into big counties, the largest of which, containing the second biggest city, Bergen, will pay any general practitioner his travelling expenses, and his locum for six weeks, in order that he may stay at a sanatorium to learn the methods of treatment there. So far this is the only county which so acts, but others are likely to follow suit soon. At least 10 per cent. of doctors have benefited by these provisions.

In the United States there seems to be considerable variation in the methods and extent of fighting tuberculosis. A good deal is still left to the efforts of voluntary charity, both in the direction of the raising of funds and the rendering of medical service by doctors. There is an energetic National Association for the Prevention of Tuberculosis, which raises a good deal of money by the sale of a special stamp. Local bodies, however, are finding more and more of the funds, and are taking an increasingly large share in organising the fight. While some municipalities concentrate more upon the work of dispensaries, town clinics, health visiting, and the publication of leaflets, others depend more upon the provision of sanatoriums or of day camps for children, and of night camps for adult workers. The segregation of infectious patients is not accomplished on a large scale. To give a concrete instance of expenditure in one of the States:—In Pennsylvania[1] up to the beginning of 1912 about six million dollars had been expended on the crusade against tuberculosis; and of this amount a little over two million was spent by private corporations, nearly three million by the Commonwealth of Pennsylvania, and about one million by the City of Philadelphia. Nearly four million of the entire amount had been expended since 1907. In 1911 there were about 1800 beds available in the Commonwealth for tuberculous cases.

In Hungary where there is obligatory sick benefit insurance for all whose salary does not exceed £100 a year, some sanatorium benefit is included. The expenses of the sick benefit fund are borne equally by employer and employed. The National Insurance fund has nothing to do with the Friendly Societies. Trades Unions have their own unemployment funds. The State makes no provision in money to the sickness or accident fund; but provides buildings, offices, and some expenses of administration. As regards sanatorium treatment, patients are sent into various parts of the country. The insurance fund pays for the railway travelling and provides free accommodation at the sanatorium for a varying length of time. But in the rural districts at all events the proportion of money spent on sanatorium treatment does not seem

[1] Lawrence, F. Flick, M.D., *Trans. Coll. Phys.*, Philadelphia, 1911.

to be high—as judged by the following figures comprising the expenditure of the total income of the Kolozsvar district :—

Sick pay	£3800
Medical Men	£1900
Payment of Officers and Administration ...	£2500
Drugs	£1200
Funeral Expenses	£700
Sanatoriums	£200
Maternity	£62

CHAPTER IV

HOW TO RAISE THE FUNDS, AND CONTROL THE EFFICIENCY OF STATE SANATORIUMS

THE different possible methods of raising a communal fund for the provision and maintenance of sanatoriums naturally coincide with the different possible authorities who may be responsible for their management and control. The fund can be raised by one or more of the following means:—

1. Voluntary charitable contributions from private individuals, generally the wealthy.

2. Direct contributions from employers of labour to ensure the better efficiency of their employees.

3. Local rates.

4. The pooled contributions of the working classes through invalidity and sickness societies, or other agencies.

5. Taxes, through the national exchequer.

Correspondingly sanatoriums can belong to any one or more of the following bodies:

1. A private person, a company, or a corporate body supported by voluntary contributions.

2. A corporate body supported by employers of labour.

3. A local authority.
4. A recognised Society, such as an approved Friendly Society, or invalidity Assurance Society.
5. A national central authority.

Now a study of the history of the gradual adoption by civilised states of the state provision of relief for the destitute, and for the sick, exhibits certain fairly well-defined tendencies. How far these tendencies can be permanently looked upon as marks of advance, remains to be seen; but it is helpful to note them. They are

1. The gradual disappearance of the efforts of voluntary charity, and their displacement by organised public relief.
2. The transition of public relief through an optional and partial stage to one of compulsory and universal application.
3. The recognition of the advisability of having, for purposes of economy and efficiency, an overseeing central authority with adequate powers of inspection and control over the local authorities, who as a rule have originally had the sole responsibility of looking after the destitute and sick.
4. The gradual disappearance of civil disabilities attaching to public relief.

In selecting the authorities for the State provision of sanatoriums, and for the supervision of the other forces under public control for fighting tuberculosis, it is well at the outset to realise fully the extent of the

battleground.   Means must be forthcoming so that
no place escapes scrutiny, and no circumstance which
contributes to the perpetuation of this disease escapes
attention.   The school, the house, the workshop, the
office, public halls and conveyances must come under
a kindly, helpful supervision.   The nursing mother,
the doctor, the health visitor, the child, the school-
teacher, the employer, the workman, the milkman, the
baker must all give and receive instruction, and have
their habits properly regulated.   And those factors contributing to the development of the disease which are
connected with wages, hours of labour, ignorance about
food values and cooking must receive due attention.
Again, any effective scheme must embrace the whole
population, whether insured persons, the dependants
of insured persons, or the uninsured.

A scheme for gradually eradicating tuberculosis
must therefore be very comprehensive ; and no part of
the scheme, not even the most important—the provision
of sanatoriums—can be sharply separated off from the
other parts.   From these considerations it follows that
a combination of authorities is to some extent not only
unavoidable, but also expedient.   At the present
moment it is not wise to attempt to define too pre-
cisely the nature of the combination required.   But
some such combined effort as that which the coming
of the Insurance Act has inaugurated will, I believe,
be found to be a good working basis.   Local government is likely in the near future to be considerably
remodelled, and the wheels of the new machinery so
recently started by the Insurance Act have as yet not
quite found how they are to fit in with previously

existing machinery, so that it would be idle to attempt to lay down final judgments on these matters. The whole subject of areas, of administrative functions of local bodies, of the inter-relation of the various authorities, of their combination in joint boards or what not, and of their connection with central departments and Parliamentary control needs the attention of politicians and thoughtful citizens. The thing ever to be borne in mind is the avoidance of waste of money and energy, by paying due regard to methods of economy, and to proper co-ordination so that over-lapping is avoided.

Help is given in the avoidance of imperfections in carrying out present and future plans not only by sensible and good combination, but also by a careful examination of any defects which have in the past been liable to occur when too much dependence has been placed upon one controlling authority.

In studying the history of the provision of sanatoriums for the people certain defects are clearly observable resulting from undue dependence upon the efforts of voluntary charity. These shortcomings are now-a-days more or less generally admitted. To summarise them, the efforts of voluntary charity generally exhibit some or all of the following defects :—(*a*) inadequacy to meet the needs arising ; (*b*) haphazard application; (*c*) a lack of proper economy; (*d*) overlapping ; and (*e*) abuse. It is because of such defects that charity is too often degrading : to quote a clever parody by Dr F. Rees[1] :—

[1] Ferdinand Rees, M.D., "National Organisation of the Profession," in *British Medical Journal*, Aug. 3rd, 1912.

"Charity is twice cursed—
It curseth him that gives and him that takes.
It puffs up the self-pride of the giver, and destroys the self-respect of the taker."

The vicarious nature of much "charity" at the expense of the medical profession is only just becoming widely and intelligently recognised by the profession. No recurrence of the following abuse of charity, for example, must be allowed in connection with the provision of sanatoriums : in the past the employers of labour have often, by their subscriptions to medical charities, bought five or six times the value of their contributions in medical comforts and maintenance for their employees. But some of the possible abuses of charity in connection with the provision of sanatoriums are more subtle. In the past many structurally fine sanatoriums have been built by philanthropists, and left without an appreciable maintenance endowment fund. The expenses of maintenance have to be met by charging patients weekly fees. Too often the philanthropy of such institutions is partly at the expense of the medical profession, because too little care is observed to keep out those patients who could afford to enter private sanatoriums run by doctors for their own living, who have started their institutions without aid from philanthropy towards initial capital charges. Again, maintenance expenses have been kept down by inadequate payment of the medical officers employed, and by under-staffing ; though this has been less detrimental to the medical profession than to the sick inmates. For the institutions have very often got only junior men without experience or incompetents.

The element of charity is best eliminated in the State provision of Sanatoriums by seeing to it that the method of raising the fund is equitable to all, that all who manage the sanatoriums are adequately remunerated, and that the standard of comfort, of living, and of medical attendance is not, in general level, above that required to meet the prevailing needs and requirements of the majority of the users of the sanatoriums.

Next, a consideration of any defects at present arising from dependence upon the rates is called for. An attempt to find an answer to the following question will be helpful :—Why is it that the fear of the rate-payer is the great hindrance to progress ? The consequent tendency to niggardliness and lack of bold measures are constantly seen where matters depend largely upon local authorities and upon the rates. I think there are, broadly, two reasons for this state of affairs. In the first place, the incidence of rating in England is inequitable. Rates fall much too much upon improvements ; they tend to hamper industry and to tax enterprise. Further, " nothing approaching uniformity or justice in the distribution of the burden of rating is anywhere to be found." National expenditure has doubled in twenty years without any appreciable popular discontent, but almost everywhere rates are felt to be burdensome. The prevalent cry of local bodies is for an increase of exchequer grants. But alteration of the basis and of the areas of rating is surely as necessary as, and probably much more necessary than, an increase in the grants from the Imperial Exchequer. In the second place local government is not as yet sufficiently in the hands of the democracy. This is perhaps especially the case in rural districts, where the labourer and small trader have little voice in local government. The democracy is perhaps still not fully awake to its responsibilities in this direction. But the people without a moderate or large amount of leisure and money generally cannot exercise much influence in local affairs because they cannot afford the time and money to participate in them. The necessity for the various representatives on the Insurance Committees, as well as on local bodies, to have at least their expenses refunded, is not recognised sufficiently widely.

I feel that the disappearance in our own country of the defects just mentioned in connection with organisations paid for out of rates and controlled by local bodies, such as Local Health Authorities, will be hastened by the creation of the new, potent authority, the Local Insurance Committee, which is developing ardour and a fresh driving force to spur all on towards the eradication of preventable disease. I believe this in spite of the fact that the Insurance Committees have not yet learned to work properly with the local bodies, to whom under the various tuberculosis notification regulations the existence of tuberculous patients is reported, and although the creation of the new authority as a separate body does not commend itself to some.

With regard to rate aid to institutions for the treatment of the sick or their dependants, there are two minor points worth attention. Firstly, there is great lack of uniformity as to how these institutions are assessed for rates. No doubt in the long run it matters little, so long as just proportions are kept, whether the rates subsidise such institutions directly, or by a combined arrangement of direct contribution and indirect subsidy through low or purely nominal assessment. But uniformity of practice in this particular seems desirable. Secondly, when the dependants of the insured become entitled to benefit under the Insurance Act, whatever example is set by State sanatoriums is likely to be followed by such other institutions as fever hospitals. At present the recipients of relief in our hospitals for such infectious diseases as scarlet fever, diphtheria etc., are for the most part treated in Municipal Hospitals free of charge, and the cost falls upon the rates.

Lastly, in this section comes the knotty subject of national subsidy and central control. On the one hand too much of either leads to the defects arising from a lessened local responsibility. Too much central control may lead to the evils of an autocratic bureaucracy, showing extravagance, pedantry, want of elasticity to varying circumstances, and a drying up of interest in, and attention to, the requirements of the nation. On the other hand experience has generally pointed to the necessity of having a certain amount of contribution from the Imperial Exchequer carrying with it central control, not only as a juster means of raising part of the funds than can otherwise be arranged, but also because some central control seems necessary to help towards the amount of uniformity consistent with efficiency, to co-ordinate things so that overlapping and waste of energy are avoided, and by various means constantly to see that efficiency and economy are followed

In this connection of economy and central control it is worth considering briefly one further point. The health insurance fund, under which sanatorium benefit comes, is directly in charge of the Treasury. It has been pointed out that the actual cost in the United Kingdom of both Old Age pensions and National Health Insurance is considerably in excess of what was originally estimated. This fact perhaps points to the inadvisability of putting the Treasury in actual charge of great spending measures. This action is something of a recent innovation. The Treasury has previously, as a rule, been a finance department acting as a guardian and as a check upon extravagance, rather than a spending department. Although it would be deplorable for the old Treasury spirit, which meant an unintelligent desire to cut down all expenditure, to creep in again ; still it does seem that there is something to be said in favour of having the Treasury a department in the State which canvasses proposed expenditure but is not a judge in its own cause.

Finally there is one good principle, not hitherto referred to, which is helpful in arranging the constitution of the various authorities, whether these be local bodies, insurance committees, federations of employers, government departments, or what not, and that is the principle of letting representation be proportionate to the contribution paid.

CHAPTER V

ON OTHER AGENCIES FOR COMBATING TUBER-
CULOSIS AND THEIR CONNECTION WITH THE
SANATORIUM

In the campaign to eradicate tuberculosis the sanatorium is only one unit, and in considering the State
provision of sanatoriums it is necessary to examine how
this unit is to fit into the general plan of the campaign.
Therefore before dealing with sanatorium construction
and management, I shall consider a few points respecting
other agencies and their connection with the sanatorium.
The most important are the tuberculosis dispensary
and the general practitioner.

Now in the first place it is expedient to recognise
fully that any schemes for combating the evils which
produce tuberculosis must be founded upon accurate
knowledge, purposefully used, and must contain everywhere the elevating influence of human sympathy. It
is no good constantly to preach the wisdom of open
windows and fresh air, without remembering at the
same time that many are unable to keep up adequate
bodily heat on account of being unable to have sufficient
food, clothing, and firing. Again, it is necessary in
some quarters to avoid converting the struggle against

tuberculosis into a war against the tuberculous. Exaggerated fears of those capable of spreading the infection, and of the infecting organism do not permit adequate comprehension of the various factors to be considered, besides tending to let a just war descend into an ill-judged persecution.

Knowledge about tuberculosis is in many particulars not yet thoroughly accurate and full. But every year makes it more complete. It is only within the last year or two that the weight of evidence from many and various sources has lead to the fairly wide acceptance, by those who are constantly studying these matters, of the following conclusions: The germs of tuberculosis are usually sown during the first years of life. By the time twelve years of age has been reached they become implanted in most of the members of an industrial, urban community, and even amongst those outside the urban districts their implantation is common in most civilised lands. The germs produce a crop of deaths within a few years of gaining access to the soil. But they produce in those who survive an acquired immunity. This immunity frequently breaks down, generally during the prime of life, and with the result that consumption develops. The break-down amongst a proportion of the population is due to bad industrial and home environment, *e.g.* defective housing, vitiated air, and low wages leading to underfeeding. More elaborate data are required relating to the incidence of consumption in various occupations, and to the influence of each of the many bad conditions of environment tending to produce the malady. The Tuberculosis Officer and the Medical Officer of Health should be mainly responsible for collecting, studying, bringing to practical use, and completing so far as possible the information about these and cognate points.

Some authorities, Dr T. D. Lister[1] for example, have recently done much to emphasise the view that the fight against tuberculosis should aim rather at eradicating the mortality and morbidity of the disease by attention to the social and industrial causes, than at exterminating the infection. True it is that removal of the infection will banish death and sickness due to the disease, but its removal is probably even more difficult to accomplish than is the attainment of the other aim ; and directing attention chiefly to the environmental causes producing the disease will do much more to help other reforms than can be expected from attacking infection alone.

The Tuberculosis Dispensary. The evidence is somewhat inconclusive that the tuberculosis death rate has been reduced by the influence of Tuberculosis Dispensaries. Although they have done something to draw attention to the evils of the old hospital out-patient system, yet exertions must still be made to counteract a present tendency to perpetuate in them the defects of that system, which generally entailed much waste of the patient's time, hurried investigation of his condition, and treatment directed merely to the relief of his symptoms, while still leaving the causes of his breakdown largely untouched. The dispensary

[1] See Dr T. D. Lister, *Daily Telegraph*, April 21st, 1913, speech at Mansion House at the annual meeting of the Hospital Saturday Fund.

must be used as a bureau for collecting, and studying the facts about the nature, growth, and distribution of the disease, and as a centre for instruction. It must be used also for purposes of diagnosis, and as a centre for co-ordinating the various forces drawn up to combat the disease. I am not a believer in using it as a centre for treatment, unless sanatorium treatment is impossible, because it leaves the patient in his original physical, emotional, and mental environment, and because, if so used, tiring and therefore injurious journeys to the dispensary are often incurred for advice, for tuberculin, or for a bottle of medicine. The medicine will probably do more harm than good; because it often does nothing but allay symptoms, and divert attention from the advice. Each dispensary should be provided with several beds into which patients may at once be taken for observation. Periodic temperature readings carefully taken while at rest for a few days constitute a most helpful aid to diagnosis. The dispensary must aid the early transference of the patient from his home to a sanatorium, and under no circumstances must it act so that the treatment at sanatoriums is deferred, or an attempt made to do without it.

Dr Leslie Mackenzie at the Tuberculosis Conference in Manchester last year[1] said, " he was inclined to think that the tuberculosis hospital would be a better starting point than the tuberculosis dispensary for treatment in the great proportion of cases, as a short period of observational treatment in hospital beds should be of the greatest value." This suggestion is met by providing the observational beds in the dispensary.

[1] *Vide British Medical Journal*, Vol. ii. p. 1372.

Eventually, perhaps, some of the dispensaries can be special departments of hospitals or infirmaries. At present, however, in the United Kingdom, Poor Law infirmaries cannot be utilised at all for any of the insured; and for this, even apart from their deficiencies, there appear to be good reasons. With regard to defects, although good special quarters for consumptives are now provided in a few infirmaries, many of these institutions are not at present suitable for dealing with the tuberculous in any way, chiefly on account of insufficient space, understaffing, and inadequacy of open windows.

Sir William Osler has been foremost in advocating that tuberculosis dispensaries should be attached to general hospitals. Certainly there are many arguments in favour of this arrangement. Tuberculosis is at present one of the commonest and most important of all diseases from which mankind suffers. It would be deplorable if the members of the staff of a general hospital were deprived, as is now too much the case, of the advantages of seeing many cases of consumption and other forms of tuberculosis. Special wards could easily be set aside, and a special department for out-patients. It would be more convenient for students to gain experience and training in respect of these patients at the general hospital to which they were attached, rather than to go to special institutions. It would perhaps also give students a better sense of the relative prevalence and importance of tuberculosis compared with other diseases if such a plan were followed. On the other hand, the teaching of fevers is in no way worse, but is perhaps better because these are treated in special hospitals. It would be easy to affiliate tuberculosis dispensaries and other institutions for the tuberculous to the teaching schools. Hospitals are at present situated for the most part in the centres of towns, which are obviously not the most ideal places for dealing with consumptives. Most probably facilities of transit will improve and ideas advance, so that before long more hospitals will be placed in the purer air of the country, but such events cannot come about in the early future.

There are two practical difficulties, which are perhaps worth mentioning, in making the tuberculosis dispensary a department of a general hospital. These have been brought to my personal attention by medical friends in two provincial towns, both of which shall be nameless. At the first a well-known officer of health was unable to make the arrangements for attaching the tuberculosis dispensary to the general hospital of the town because the hospital staff were jealous of one another. They felt that it was not possible for them all to serve in the special department, and that if one of their number was appointed for this purpose, he would thereby gradually gain the consulting practice with regard to cases of tuberculosis in the town and neighbourhood. They could not contemplate such a possibility with equanimity. In the other important provincial town the step of attaching a tuberculosis dispensary to the general hospital had already been taken, but the tuberculosis officer—a man of considerable acumen and experience—was often bitter in his complaints as to how hampered he was by the interference and ignorance of the staff in his special subject.

Now with respect to the *general practitioner*, no scheme should fail to procure for everyone—well or ill—a home doctor ; not necessarily, however, a doctor who will treat the individual patient when ill—especially perhaps if ill from any form of tuberculosis. The exact part to be played by a sanatorium doctor, namely to treat the sick and to instruct the convalescent, seems immediately clear. But the parts which the general practitioner, the medical officer of health, and the special tuberculosis officer respectively have to play are at present somewhat indefinite, and are likely to remain ambiguous and variable until certain transitions have occurred. At the present moment it is still all too true that a great many practitioners are ill-grounded in the fundamental principles underlying the early diagnosis and proper treatment of tuberculosis. Again most medical officers of health are experienced more in administration than in clinical work, or at all events they have not as a rule any extensive training in treating those with lung disease. And the number of thoroughly competent tuberculosis officers is admittedly too few. The majority of general practitioners apparently has not yet grasped the probable trend of events. For last year our British Medical Association, although many of the claims it put forward were quite sound[1], in its efforts to forward an anti-tuberculosis scheme in accordance with the Government's plan and with its own wishes, seemed frightened of change, and too apprehensive of doing damage to the welfare of the private practitioner, remunerated by the sick according to visits paid. And plenty of practitioners are to be

[1] *Vide British Medical Journal*, 1912, Vol. II. p. 392.

found bemoaning that soon there will be nothing left for them to do, when, to quote from a general practitioner's recent letter to the press, "the Public Health Department have robbed us of most of our infectious cases; the educational authorities are threatening to provide their children with medical treatment; the State is appointing whole-time officers to man tubercular dispensaries, where tubercular cases will be treated."

Already the medical profession is recognising that this kind of medical work is still being done by practitioners in the science and art of medicine, and at rates of remuneration approaching the reasonable and adequate. And before long doctors will come also to see that the general practitioner of the future will be more of a preventer, a diagnoser, and a teacher of hygiene than he is at present; and less of a man somewhat vainly attempting to cope with conditions he can but ill control, and to cure disease after it has broken out rampantly. The transition stage from the one to the other has already been reached in England, for under the tuberculosis scheme of the Insurance Act it seems likely that by degrees the general practitioner will be called upon to look after the home condition of the patient and of those who come in contact with him, and to supervise the "aftercare" of the convalescent. In this scheme care is being taken, or will soon be taken, to see that there is no postponement in consulting a doctor, no unreasonable delay in arriving at a diagnosis, no omission of good arrangements for examining contacts, and no lack of all the requisites for proper supervision and treatment at home, during the stages when such a course seems desirable or necessary. In this scheme the medical officer of health, the tuberculosis officer, and the general practitioner must each bear his part : the first as co-ordinator and general administrative adviser; the second probably filling the place of consultant diagnostician, examiner of contacts, and adviser as to the best line of treatment to adopt ; while the third, probably aided by a nurse, will chiefly be concerned in looking after the home conditions. Both the general practitioner and the nurse will be in close touch on the one hand with the members of the District Insurance Committee, many of whom, no doubt by voluntary effort, can render a useful part in this connection ; and on the other hand with the tuber-culosis officer; while the latter must work in friendly co-operation with the medical officer of health and with the sanatorium doctor. Finally, the duty of these various medical men to collaborate in keeping useful records must be mentioned. These records will form an integral part of the statistics and information upon the health of insured persons, which is a duty imposed upon the Insurance Committees.

CHAPTER VI

THE CONSTRUCTION OF A STATE SANATORIUM

GOOD reasons for looking upon the site of a sanatorium as a plague spot in the neighbourhood in which it is situated, are conspicuous by their absence. Consumption is an infective disease, in that it is one produced by the invasion of a known micro-organism, the tubercle bacillus. But it is not infectious in the sense in which that word is usually understood. It is not spread in like manner to scarlet fever, measles, small-pox, etc. A well-conducted sanatorium and its neighbourhood can be looked upon as one of the safest and most salubrious places possible, for there fresh, pure country air and sunshine invade all the buildings and grounds, and every one of the simple precautions necessary is taken, such as the proper disposal of the sputum.

The site of a sanatorium is not of the foremost importance, so long as practical considerations of the expense of capital outlay and of maintenance are always borne in mind. Too often ease of getting good water supply, of maintaining proper disposal of sewage and slop-water, expense of cartage, facility of transit of patients, and such matters are forgotten in striving after the acquisition of a site with the best possible aspect and shelter, and in the most salubrious air. An aspect facing S.S.E. is best in this country. It is better than one facing due S. or S.W.; for the commonest wind is a south-westerly one, and this, too, is the prevalent rainy wind; whereas an easterly wind or even a S.E. one is comparatively rare in every part of the country. Further, morning sun shining into a room is preferable to evening sun. This is especially so in warm weather, when the former allows the room to cool down nicely before night; also sunblinds are then unnecessary. A suitable site would be one which sloped south and was protected from northerly winds. The buildings should be placed away from the dust of the road and surrounded by gardens and walks. The grounds should be ample enough to provide opportunity for whatever graduated labour may be prescribed for patients. The ideal situation, difficult to find, for a sanatorium for the working classes, is in a neighbourhood free from public houses, and one where open spaces of commons or woods allow plenty of scope for rambling, a great blessing to the more stalwart patients.

Sanatoriums are likely to be wanted for many a day. The knowledge of the best kind of architectural arrangement for an institution of this sort has now reached a stage when it is worth while to build in a material of a more lasting nature than wood, or other cheap material. The opinion that it is necessary to destroy periodically such a building for hygienic reasons is incorrect. Due cleanliness and periodic, thorough disinfection are all that is necessary. Therefore it is a distinct advantage to construct the sanatorium of substantial materials, such as brick and plaster. Such a plan, however, costs more than building of an inexpensive material. By the following means, however, the expense of the initial outlay can be kept low: (*a*) by keeping the height of rooms down to reasonable dimensions ; (*b*) by building in several places three, and in other places two, storeys under one roof ; (*c*) by avoiding the necessity for any appreciable number of shelters, useful adjuncts though they be ; and (*d*) by so planning things that expenditure on furnishing, especially as to the provision of long-chairs, can be kept low. It is false economy to keep the price of construction down too low. At least £170 per bed inclusive ought to be allowed, and probably by a skilful attention to the above points this sum would be sufficient to allow substantial materials to be used where the number of beds is 130 or over.

I have arrived at the above conclusions, and those about to be mentioned, after considerable experience, first as a sanatorium patient, then for several years as a sanatorium doctor and manager, and after helpful and repeated conference with three persons pre-eminent in the British Isles amongst those who have had experience in the practical management of sanatoriums for the working classes, namely Dr Jane Walker, Dr Esther Carling and Mr Carling. They have been carried through, as far as the designs (at end of book), after consultation between the firm of Messrs Percy Adams, Holden, and Pearson, well-known and experienced hospital and sanatorium architects, and myself.

The height of a not over large room need not, for

purposes of proper ventilation or for æsthetic reasons, be above $8\frac{1}{2}$ feet on the ground floor, and either $8\frac{1}{2}$ feet or even 8 feet above this. When the height of rooms is not excessive, much material is saved, stairs need not be steep, and lifts are unnecessary, especially when no patient's room is placed higher than the first floor above the ground floor.

If the patients' bedrooms are skilfully planned so as to be conveniently used for day resting places, whether the patient is quite ill or well forward in convalescence, there is no necessity for provision of revolving or other forms of shelters, liegehalle, verandahs, balconies, or long chairs. Against some of these things there are several sound arguments besides the important one of increased expense. The following reason for providing a few shelters exists; it is of educational advantage to teach people to sleep out in a shelter after leaving the sanatorium. Shelters are sometimes provided in patient's own homes by local bodies when large window space and sufficient floor space are not there procurable. Till better housing conditions can be brought about such provision is sometimes of undoubted help, otherwise it would be inadvisable to run the risk of allowing it tacitly to be thought necessary to provide something of a special nature. If a few shelters are built at a sanatorium they should not be extras, but should form part of the sleeping accommodation for convalescents.

Balconies are objectionable on the following grounds :

1. They are detrimental to quiet and privacy ;

2. They diminish light and air in the rooms ;

3. They collect wet, and consequently are apt to rot woodwork ;

4. They make it difficult to maintain protection against some winds and at the same time an abundance of fresh air.

Although balconies have some advantages, the balance is heavily against them.   Similarly, many of the same arguments apply to a verandah.   If it is glass-covered, special contrivances costing extra money have to be provided to avoid undue heat when the sun is shining brightly.   If it is of a solid material it shuts out light. If it faces in a southerly direction, then it is neither pleasant nor desirable to use when a strong wind is blowing from any such quarter.

In order that a room may be not only a good one for a patient when in bed, but also a convenient, pleasant, desirable, and efficient place for a convalescent to rest in during the day-time, the following points are necessary :

1. Fresh air must be abundant whatever the direction of the wind, yet as far as possible when a high wind is blowing from any quarter of the compass the room must not be wind-swept.

2. A patient lying on his bed must be able to see out of a window or door.

3. The room must be so arranged that the bed naturally stands so that neither side is directly against a wall.

4. Every room must at some time or other of the day receive at least a little sunlight, and so far as possible in the climate of the United Kingdom those

rooms used by patients confined, or chiefly confined, to bed should have an aspect mainly southerly.

5. No patient must at night be within close proximity and consequent easy hearing of many others, otherwise the difficulty of sleeplessness caused by a neighbour's cough may arise.

6. Every batch of rooms must have adequate and handy washing and bathing arrangements available, also if possible a drying room for patients' clothes, and adequate space for closets, linen, boots, etc.

Other points of importance in connection with the arrangements of patients' rooms are :

1. Separation of the sexes, whether fellow patients or patients and attendants, must be planned as strictly as possible in any sanatorium for the working classes of both sexes.

2. The sick should be placed in a separate block, or well away from the convalescents. Even if a sanatorium is solely for slight cases, provision must always be made for at least a proportion of people confined to bed. This part of the building should have easy access to both kitchen and nurses' quarters, and be well away from the recreation room.

With respect to other architectural features in the planning of a State provided sanatorium the following are a few points to note :

1. Heating appliances are unnecessary in this climate for the majority of patients' bedrooms. But economy of heat, of pipes, and other heating appliances must be constantly borne in mind in planning the whole scheme of a sanatorium.

2. The quarters of the doctors, secretary, and matron, or at least of some or other of such officers must, for purposes of discipline, have a position capable of inspiring a feeling of good supervision.

3. Servants' quarters must be well away from patients' quarters.

The plans (at end of book) are for a sanatorium of 150 to 250 beds. From a medical point of view an institution of this size is too large, because the head doctor cannot give the individual attention which is desirable to the study of so many patients. But local authorities have to study economy, and at present smaller sanatoriums will often be impracticable, especially when the number for whom provision may have to be made is considered. About a quarter of a million persons in the United Kingdom are entitled to sanatorium benefit; but up to April 30th of this year (1913) not quite a tenth of this number had applied for it. Soon, however, it is to be hoped that matters will move more quickly in all directions in connection with sanatorium provision and benefit.

Besides conforming to the principles detailed above the plans as above exhibit the following arrangements and advantages:

(1) The Resident Medical Officer's House is away from the main building with a private garden not overlooked by patients, but the windows of the house command the grounds to some extent to ensure the supervision of patients.

(2) Assistant R.M.O.'s are provided with rooms in the Administration Block.

(3) Nurses' quarters, including quarters for Matron and Housekeeper, are provided in the upper part of the Administration Block, with a separate entrance and staircase. An alternative arrangement would be to place the nurses in a separate " home " with a private garden, at the same time providing rooms for night nurses near to the bedrooms for the sick.

(4) The Administration Block contains an Entrance Hall, Waiting Room, Consulting Room, small Operating Room for throat examinations, dentistry, etc., Dispensary, Laboratory, Secretary's, Steward's and assistant R.M.O.'s rooms.

(5) The Dining Hall and Recreation Rooms are placed in a central position.

(6) The Kitchen Block is in connection with the Dining Hall and also has easy access to the Sick Patients' Block.

The Kitchen is top-lighted and well ventilated ; opening out of it are sculleries for washing-up and for vegetables. Between the Kitchen and Dining Room is a Servery fitted with hot-plates, etc., and a pantry fitted with teak sink. There should be a separate pantry or washing-up arrangement for the Nurses and Staff.

In connection with the Kitchen are a Servants' Hall, Sewing Room, Linen Store, Housekeeper's Office and Store, Meat and Milk Larders facing north, and ample Coal Stores. On the upper floors are the Servants' Bedrooms.

(7) The Laundry and Boiler House is placed away from the sanatorium in such a position that the prevailing wind does not carry smoke and dust from

the chimney shaft into the patients' quarters. In connection with this block are the Disinfector and the Mortuary. Sputum can be burned in the boiler furnaces.

(8) The Patients' Blocks are split up into Pavilions:

(*a*) For Sick Patients: in these blocks many patients, but not all, have a separate room (about 12' 0" × 10' 0") facing south with a corridor on the north, out of which open lobbies to sanitary annexes, staircases, etc. Many patients amongst the insured object strongly to sleeping in a room alone; sometimes because they imagine they are so ill that they are likely to die. Therefore some double-bedded rooms, and a few wards for more than two, are provided.

Every patient is provided with a cupboard in the bedroom, 3' 0" wide, 1' 3" deep, consisting of hanging space for clothes with a shelf over.

(*b*) For Ambulant Patients: in these blocks patients are placed in wards divided into sections by partitions and doors: the latter can be opened back during the day. The space per patient in an ordinary hospital ward is about 1350 cub. feet, but in a sanatorium, where the windows are large and open to the full extent with a consequent decrease in the height of the ward, a space per patient of 750 cub. feet is sufficient. There would be no washstands in these wards, but a separate Sanitary Annex is provided, cut off by a cross-ventilated lobby. There is provision in this annex for douche-baths (1 to every 8 patients) with dressing spaces, a long bath, towel drying rails, shelves for hot-water bottles, drying room for wet clothes, boot room with seats, racks, and bench for cleaning; water and earth closets (1 to every 8 patients); sink room and linen store.

The plan of a section of the block for ambulant patients shows; (i) How each patient can at night time be shut off from all the other patients save three. (ii) How ample and free air can reach the region of every patient's bed, even should a high wind from one side necessitate the closing up of all the windows and doors on that side. A small amount of movement of the air keeps it clean and fresh, and is therefore beneficial, but it is detrimental for a patient to be placed actually in a wind. (iii) How advantageously everything is planned to permit of the beds being suitably used as places for resting on in the day time. A few old newspapers to obviate the necessity for removing boots from the feet, and a back-rest on the bed, made with but slight expense of canvas and a wooden frame, are then all that is necessary for comfort and efficiency. By these means the expense of duplicating a rest place for each patient by providing a long chair and a revolving, or other less efficient and pleasant form of shelter, is obviated.

A duty room for the nurse is sometimes required in the block for Ambulant Patients. It should be in a central position. When it is not required for this use it can be utilised for a patient. A small room for the sputum flasks and cups should be placed in a convenient central position for each of the patients' blocks. These arrangements are convenient for teaching every patient a simple plan of cleansing the cups and flasks.

The Patients' Blocks should be two storeys in height and the ground floor should be raised above the ground at least three feet with a ventilated space beneath. The windows must come either down to the floor or the sills must be kept low, say two feet from the floor, so that patients may see out. In some positions windows of the railway carriage type are convenient. They have the following advantages : full air space, or any required amount of intermediate protection between being widely open and completely shut ; no creaking ; no banging ; and no breaking.

The raising of the ground-floor is advisable to avoid ground dampness and mists, and to ensure ventilation under all floors. This plan is healthier, and in the long run economical to the building structures. Furthermore patients, especially female patients, often have strong prejudices against sleeping on, or close to the ground level, when windows or doors are open down to the floor. Privacy when undressing is not so readily obtained, and the entrance of rats and of other animals is feared.

The materials depend on the amount of money available and partly on the locality, but they should be as far as possible hard, impervious and free from joints. Such materials as bricks, reinforced concrete, cement, tiles, etc., are suitable, and all internal angles should be rounded when expense permits and all mouldings omitted. In the case of timber all wood-work exposed to the weather should be treated with creosote or other such mixture to save painting, and all floors should be freely ventilated so that linoleum may be put down at any point.

CHAPTER VII

THE PRINCIPLES TO BE FOLLOWED IN MANAGING
A STATE SANATORIUM

CONSIDERATION of the more important matters connected with the management of a State Sanatorium fall naturally under the two heads: doctor, and patient. But first there are a few matters of a general nature, and the most important of these is the question of the cost of maintenance. The estimate for this depends partly upon the size of the sanatorium and upon the stage of the disease of the majority of the inmates. If the institution contains a large proportion of severe and advanced cases, the annual maintenance cost per bed should not be less than 32*s*. weekly. Otherwise, this may be reduced to about 28*s*. weekly. Experience in Germany seems to show that the immediate cost to sickness funds is greater the more institutional treatment is depended upon in contradistinction to treatment at home. But in this respect a sanatorium, where the remedial measures are inexpensive, should set a good example; for in the methods of conducting other similar institutions a tendency to over-emphasise the importance of elaborate means of treatment (such as vaccines, expensive drugs, X-rays, etc.), is often much in evidence.

Now *the sanatorium doctor* must be an autocrat. His powers must not be unduly curtailed by any committee. Otherwise discipline, so necessary to be kept up strictly, and often so difficult to maintain in a sanatorium for the working classes, cannot be kept. Yet some young physicians, when they become sanatorium doctors, may use the powers they find themselves in possession of, without tact, and without due regard to the interests of the sick worker. The sanatorium doctor must learn to use his powers aright, and to co-operate properly with the medical officers, and the committees, with whom he finds himself labouring, or under whose ægis his services are rendered.

When the State undertakes the provision of sanatorium treatment for tuberculosis, the amount of personal attention required from the doctor of the institution must be ample. What is considered ample at present may soon be thought to be inadequate. Sanatoriums of 150 to 250 beds are now contemplated, or are already in existence. For such an institution three (or four) doctors are considered sufficient. But the essence of recent advances in medical treatment is the appreciation of the necessity for close personal supervision. This is seen particularly in connection with those suffering from mental ailments, where the methods of psycho-analysis make great demands upon the time and patience of the physician; and to a less extent in connection with the supervision of the remedial measures and of the proper training of the individual in hygiene, in the case of Phthisis. I believe, therefore, that a good arrangement to aim at in the management of State sanatoriums is that of having an institution where the maximum number of patients is 75. Then one head doctor with two assistants can study sufficiently closely all the patients under his care.

The arrangements made for staffing State sanatoriums and dispensaries, etc., with medical officers must avoid the slightest continuance of that present wrong system, seen particularly in the case of our hospitals, by which a few great indirect rewards received by the staff are set off against a vast mass of almost compulsory almsgiving by the rank and file of the profession. These indirect rewards, too, viz. experience, advertisement, and honour must be more widely spread amongst the whole body of the medical profession. Already owing to the National Insurance Act good steps are being taken towards breaking down such anomalous evils as these, and others which are all too rife at the present day in the arrangements of medical services in the United Kingdom. And this improvement is particularly evident on the side of " Sanatorium Benefit"; except perhaps in so far as concerns the spread of experience, where organisation is distinctly incomplete. Adequate and direct remuneration for medical services rendered lies at the root of this question ; for if the remuneration is both adequate and direct, evils of this kind are not usually present, nor likely to creep in. In some ways it is ridiculous that a salary of £500 or £600 should be considered the right one for the chief medical officer and manager of a large, complicated, and important medical institution like a sanatorium for 150 or more patients ; yet at the present moment it seems to be not only the one which the public considers adequate, but also that which a majority of the profession considers just.   I hope that the day is at hand when the public appreciation of the importance of health will be such as to demand and get many men worthy of earning considerably higher salaries, and that the public will then be able, as I have little doubt, to get also its money's-worth.

The sanatorium patient cannot be only he who is suffering from quite slight manifestations of tuberculosis.   Sometimes a so-called "early case" turns out to be one whose outlook is bad, and *vice versa*.   Cases indeterminate for purposes of such classification are common.   Pathologically the really early case of phthisis in an adult is probably one of the rarities of medicine; for more knowledge is revealing that phthisis is generally acquired long before the occurrence of symptoms demonstrating its presence.   In fact many hold, and on good grounds, that the seeds of consumption in the majority of cases first take root during the early years of childhood.   Great difficulties remain to be surmounted in order to get those with early symptoms into sanatoriums, in spite of the better examination of contacts, and in spite of the provision of sustenance funds for dependants.

People in England are sometimes biassed against entering a sanatorium, a place where the visitor can usually be discriminated by his wan and pale aspect from the robust looking patients.   Some seem to think that if recourse must be had to a sanatorium the condition of the patient is hopeless.   Others have a queer idea of what life in a sanatorium is like.   Again many are ignorant of the importance of comparatively slight lapses from health. Doctors, although much better educated in such matters than formerly, still occasionally fail even to suspect consumption when confronted by such symptoms as indigestion, persistent lassitude of vague origin, unaccountable loss of weight, strength, or appetite, or progressive anaemia—all common symptoms of the malady. Valuable time is often lost until such symptoms as night sweats and cough present themselves, especially when definite physical signs of the disease remain obscure, or undiscovered. The detection of the early signs in the chest is a matter of delicacy: it is usually beyond the powers of the inexperienced, and is often quite difficult even to the expert. The old fashioned idea of giving the patient the benefit of the doubt consisted in refusing to diagnose phthisis unless the signs were beyond question. The new fashion will be the reverse of this, because it will be learnt that the treatment of the debility, manifested by one symptom or another, in a sanatorium will always be advantageous to the individual.

If sanatoriums are kept only for slight cases, what is to become of the advanced, and the moderately advanced ones? The problem of the provision of suitable places for the latter remains, even if the strong disinclination of the former to go into special institutions be overcome. These institutions are liable to become labelled "homes for the dying." The difficulty of getting the advanced consumptive to accede to isolation, especially far from his relatives and friends, is experienced in most countries,—in Germany and in the States, for example.

4—2

For such reasons, therefore, where a comparatively small number of consumptives have to be dealt with, it is best to place all together. When large numbers are being arranged for, and economy demands a good deal of grouping, probably the best plan is to have two slightly different classes of sanatoriums;—one within easy reach of thickly populated centres with a somewhat larger staff of nurses, ward-men, or ward-maids, etc., than the other type possesses; to this all patients are at first sent. The other, situated in the more remote country, is utilised by drafting those convalescents into it who are able to take plentiful exercise, or graduated labour. Then two tendencies, both liable to occur in sanatoriums, can be countered by balancing the one against the other. On the one hand some, without thought or wisdom, counting the measure and indications of progress as equivalent to the progress itself, are for ever attempting to incite their physician to push them on to higher grades of exercise. The influence of these usually makes it easy, therefore, to get patients to undertake good walks, or " work in the garden," so soon as they are really ready for these stages. On the other hand, in a sanatorium for the workers, sometimes the tendency is found for lazy inmates to hanker after remaining in the institution where they have to fend for themselves but little as to domestic duties. Again, this plan may help to some extent to get over the difficulty of segregating those with advanced disease, a difficulty some day to be partly overcome by utilising for such patients beds set free in our centrally situated town hospitals and infirmaries by the removal from them of the more chronic cases into country institutions.

I agree with the conclusions of the Astor Departmental Committee on Tuberculosis as to the methods of dealing with children having tuberculosis, and with those suffering from "surgical" tuberculosis.

With regard to compulsion : Universal compulsory notification of tuberculosis is now rightly accepted in the United Kingdom. The uses made of notification are not necessarily those hitherto found advisable in dealing with other notifiable diseases. The notification of the zymotic fevers (scarlet fever, small-pox, etc.) at once suggests to the public ideas of isolation, segregation, and disinfection. In the case of tuberculosis notification must be used more for the study of the facts regarding the disease than for these other purposes. With regard to compulsory segregation : however advantageous to the individual and to the community may be the acquisition of compulsory powers for sending a patient to an institution, or for keeping him in one, the time is not yet ripe for the enactment of such powers, except so far as concerns some advanced consumptives capable of being proved a serious danger to others. Possibly increased education may render the establishment of such powers by law unnecessary. Lastly under this head comes the subject of disciplinary powers in sanatoriums. These should be vested in the chief doctor, and should include the power of the dismissal of a patient. Since, however, the loss of benefits resulting from dismissal may be heavy, the discretion of the doctor in the exercise of his powers can reasonably be subject to appeal to such a committee as the Insurance Act sets up for such circumstances. Such committees generally behave reasonably, and are disposed to uphold the authority of those in posts of responsibility. Of course, any matter which is purely medical should be referred, if occasion arise, to a purely professional tribunal. Purely medical matters connected with treatment, too, should be left solely to the sanatorium doctor, aided perhaps by advice, but not hampered by interference, from a medical advisory board or committee. Such an arrangement ought to make secure that no form of specific treatment is established, the efficacy of which has not been proved beyond question. Some medical board or committee of this kind will take over the supervision of research, and an arrangement of this sort is outlined in the recent final report of the Astor Departmental Committee.

CHAPTER VIII

THE ADVANTAGES OF SANATORIUM TREATMENT
OVER DOMICILIARY

THE State provision of sanatoriums is worthy to be given foremost place in the campaign against tuberculosis only because it is likely to influence in a more far-reaching way than anything else the evils which are going on steadily in the homes of the people, and to a certain extent elsewhere. The controllable causes of disease are for the most part those due to bad conditions of environment, and to improper personal hygiene. It is becoming recognised that hereditary causes are of much less importance than was once surmised ; and only seldom is it desirable or possible to control them. In the case of tuberculosis they are virtually negligible. The attempt to eradicate tuber- culosis, largely by attention to a correct mode of life in the individual members of society, necessitating incidentally good environment, will help forward the progress of many other social reforms. The cure of the patient in a sanatorium is, then, in some ways of secondary importance to the influence which his education has upon all with whom he comes in contact. And this influence is exerted not alone in preventing tuberculosis, but also in helping to banish other preventable diseases, and in aiding the advance of other social reforms. The superior efficacy of sanatorium treatment over domiciliary from the curative point of view is definite and decided, as I hope now to demonstrate; but sanatorium treatment is also more efficient than is treatment at home in the preventive and educational directions. With the latter subject I shall deal in the second half of this chapter.

Although the curative measures upon which the treatment of the tuberculous depends are for the most part simple in nature, the essential thing about them is thoroughness. The facilities, inducements, and forces which aid the patient to keep performing for a long space of time the little things which are of such great importance in the cure of the tuberculous, are greater in a sanatorium than at home. To perseverance and thoroughness is to be added time as necessary to bring about recovery. A week or two in a sanatorium is not of much good from a curative point of view. Three months should be looked upon as a minimum. Amongst the many better facilities aiding the cure one not very obvious one is that obtained through the moral influence of grouping the people who are striving after the same end. Being actuated by a common desire, they pool their personalities, as it were, and help one another's progress. The treatment of a sick person at home as a rule interferes with the work of healthy people. Further, a consumptive is generally a lonely invalid at home, surrounded by healthy people who are more likely to hinder than to help his progress, however much they may desire the contrary. The patient can be taught more quickly in a sanatorium than at home that his life depends upon the thoroughness of the teaching he receives, and of his acquisition thereof. Again, by the precepts of the doctors and nurses in constant attendance, and through the drilled example and common knowledge of fellow patients, he learns more quickly than he could at home the rules of hygiene which are to save his life and keep his health restored. Also he learns to gauge aright the seriousness of the disease from which he is suffering; and this is not only difficult, but also most important in helping to bring about and maintain a cure. This difficulty is easy to realise when it is remembered that a moderate number of those with early symptoms do not feel ill, that many soon reach a stage of convalescence when they feel better than they have done for years, and that with some the proverbial "spes phthisica" is prominent, while others too readily give themselves over to serious depression. In a sanatorium there is no temptation for the patient to attempt to follow his occupation at all, so that he can devote himself to his health alone. The sanatorium doctors and nurses have more specialised knowledge and expert experience than can be provided under domiciliary treatment.

On the other side a few arguments can be found which at first sight seem to favour domiciliary treatment. There is, for example, less expense to sickness funds if institutional treatment is not relied upon too much. But the cheap does not here, I believe, in the long run mean the economical. Again, sickness benefit is sometimes forfeited when an insured beneficiary goes into an institution. But this is of no moment unless he or she has dependants, and under such circumstances arrangements are now generally made for the dependants to receive the benefit. Some think, too, that the teaching of the rules of hygiene can be more direct in the home, where the faults of environment and personal conduct can be pointed out on the spot. But in my belief, the important "details" can be carried out and taught much more thoroughly and quickly by a few weeks in a sanatorium than by a much longer period under domiciliary treatment, even though the help of an excellent nurse and an able doctor, aided by the advice of a tuberculosis officer, is obtained. Again, there is in sanatorium treatment the danger of fostering valetudinarianism. But if this danger is constantly borne in mind it can generally be coped with fairly easily.

The cure of the patient is certainly hastened by his removal from the manifold deleterious influences of his home surroundings, which are rife even in the homes of those with ample means. Various home defects can, no doubt, be made good; but seldom can all be overcome. How manifold and deleterious those influences are, and how much more efficacious sanatorium treatment is than domiciliary, have already been indicated, but both can be emphasised and a few further points brought out by briefly going through seriatim some essential features of the treatment:

REST. Every consumptive patient must at some period of treatment have plenty of rest. Apart from bodily rest, rest to the mind is of importance. Now in most households bodily, and mental rest are not easily obtained ; certainly not in those of the working classes. Yet they can be procured easily in a sanatorium. Again, the degree of rest must be graded according to the patient's condition. Absolute and long continued rest in bed is sometimes required. The gradations of rest can be better prescribed and carried out in a sanatorium than at home, not only because of better facilities, but also because the supervision is closer and more skilful.

FOOD. The majority of artisans are ignorant of food values and cooking. Few housewives and fewer men amongst the working classes know how to cook even the plainest food, or what to take or avoid. Alcohol is commonly abused. There can be no doubt that the chances of making a recovery, and of making it as quickly as possible, are much greater on account of these factors being better looked after in a sanatorium than they can be under the best circumstances of most homes.

AIR. Similar remarks apply to the procuring of fresh air. At a sanatorium there is no overcrowding, and there is no undue shutting of windows. Each patient has as much space, and as much fresh air as are necessary.

EXERCISE. The exercise which must alternate with the rest as soon as all traces of fever have gone must be very carefully graduated, and this is easier to do and to supervise in a sanatorium than it is at home.

Mental influences are all important in effecting a cure. It is necessary sometimes, for example, to apply the close supervision obtained in an institution to prevent the production of that class of individual of whom it can be literally said, "He enjoys poor health." Every doctor of experience knows how important it is in the treatment of a patient to get to know the man, and to influence any temperamental peculiarities which may be detrimental to progress. This is especially true in the case of anyone suffering from a malady of a chronic nature, and it is certainly easier to accomplish in a sanatorium than at home. Again, in a sanatorium usually every mental influence is calculated to be helpful. Encouragement and cheerfulness can be turned on and kept on in a sanatorium as much as may be required. Sanatoriums may be depressing to healthy outsiders. To patients they are not so. At home quite often relatives are over anxious and depressing in their very anxiety to be cheering, especially if things are not going as well as possible.

Sometimes a patient is inclined to find the routine of treatment irksome. In that case following the régime in the company of others in a properly conducted institution is most helpful. The importance of good mental influences is well brought out by two sentences written by Dr Jane Walker a few years ago: "The qualities which most aid consumptives in recovery are, firstly: strength of will; secondly: common sense; and thirdly: equability of temperament. Therefore the essentials in the treatment of consumption are to preserve and strengthen the physique, to enforce prudence, and to induce placidity." To develop these qualities where they exist only in the germ is often impossible under home conditions, yet much deficiency in these particulars can be made up under institutional régime. Again, life in a sanatorium precludes all coddling. Long tradition has erroneously instilled into the minds of the people that coddling is of prime importance in the treatment of any complaint. Coddling is especially bad in the case of consumption.

Moral influences are closely allied to the mental and to matters of temperament, and one or two demand brief attention. One argument often brought against institutional treatment by those who speak in favour of home treatment is, that it is not good for the family to be relieved of the nursing of a sick member; that it loosens family responsibility. "One suspects that the users of this argument believe that some families are glad to get rid of their sick; of course it is the other way, it is a greater hardship for a family to let one of its members go to a sanatorium and so be separated from them. No one would think of entrusting a surgical operation to the family, yet consumption is as serious a matter as most operations. 'But, of course it would be under the close supervision of a doctor,' they say, 'and the family would only be carrying out his orders'; but consumption is too serious a matter for amateurs, however willing. Every single advantage is wanted[1]." The strain of the illness of a dear one must not be rendered unendurable, nor even too disconcerting, yet the moral gain to be obtained by a certain amount of strain must not be entirely lost. It seems to me this result is secured by recourse to institutional treatment.

Vaccines, or other similar remedies are best administered in a sanatorium. The more knowledge there is gained of the workings of the human machine, the more intricate and wonderful is found to be the machinery. And amongst the most intricate qualities can be placed those connected with immunity. Now-a-days there is in many quarters a fashion of talking glibly of auto-inoculations in connection with the treatment of tuberculosis, as if the processes underlying the ideas grouped under this term were of quite a simple nature. These processes are not simple. The same is true of the processes underlying hetero-inoculation, that is the processes involved in the attempt to bring about immunity against disease by means of administering dead bacteria or the products of bacteria cultivated and concocted outside the human body. In both cases, with respect to tuberculosis at all events, further knowledge reveals the necessity for close study and precision not only of the means used, but also of the methods of using them, and of the exact conditions of the patient when they are being used. Again, if home treatment comprises amongst other things the administration of tuberculin, a false sense of security is

[1] D. L. Cameron, *British Journal of Tuberculosis*, p. 101, April, 1913.

apt to be given to a patient; for he believes, especially if he gets on well when having it, that he is receiving treatment which is alone adequate for his cure, and thereby he may be led to slur over the rules of hygienic living which are essential for him to learn. Such a course too, I fear, rather frequently results either in the production of a chronic or of an acute disease, both of which may be very difficult to cure. Such cases provide the majority of bacilli carriers.

Cleanliness, etc. The details of clothing, and of bathing, and, most important of all, of instruction in the full meaning of the word infection, and in the means of avoiding both self-infection and the infection of others, are all factors which influence recovery. These details and this instruction are better carried out under sanatorium régime than they can be at home.

When the results of treatment from a curative point of view are looked at, institutional treatment carried on by resident experts, especially where these institutions are well staffed, bears excellent comparison with domiciliary, or with the treatment in hospitals where the residents are junior men without experience, supervised by a non-resident visiting staff. This is especially observable in the case of the special institutions for tuberculous disease of bones and joints[1]. But the same is to be found in connection with sanatoriums for consumption. This is only what is to be expected when the advantages are realised fully of having doctors who have devoted years to the special study of the disease they are treating, who reside with

---

[1] *Vide* R. C. Elmslie, *Lancet*, Feb. 17, 1912, p. 425.

their patients and are constantly supervising their lives and treatment.

The Educational Influence of Sanatoriums

The educational influence of sanatoriums can be seen by a study of how the chief factors causing tuberculosis are affected by these institutions; and the superiority in this direction of sanatorium treatment over treatment at home, thereby immediately becomes apparent. The factors of first importance causing tuberculosis are :

(A)　The absence of clean air, especially in bed-rooms and work-rooms.

(B)　The presence of the tubercle bacillus.

(C)　The poor means hitherto existent for ensuring an early diagnosis and for the adequate treatment of the disease.

(D)　Certain social and industrial conditions affecting the food and work of the individual.

(A)　*The absence of clean air.* The sanatorium treatment of consumption first raised hopes of the possibility of curing the individual and of ridding mankind of the scourge. The birth and spread of these hopes antedated Koch's great discovery of the tubercle bacillus. Their basis was the appreciation of the necessity for clean air to breathe. The influence of sanatoriums upon spreading an appreciation of this necessity remains pre-eminent.

How much there is still to do in teaching the necessity for clean air everywhere is shown on all sides. Progress will be slow so long as the professional classes, the architects, doctors, lawyers, legislators and teachers allow public buildings to be so badly ventilated as most now are. Delegates and doctors met in conference not long ago during the hottest time of summer under the auspices of the "National Association for the Prevention of Consumption" in a hall incapable of having its effete air replenished. Open air schools are being used more and more. Yet in many places new National Schools are being built having plenty of window space and sunny aspect, but with comparatively little of it available, and usually less of it utilised for the changing of the much used internal air. What is the sense of giving lessons in hygiene, including the necessity for fresh air, when the child is compelled to spend many hours a day in the unsavoury atmosphere of an ill-ventilated, over-crowded schoolroom? Much used air is polluted air. People should as lief breathe polluted air as drink polluted water. Windows are made for air as well as light. No satisfactory means of ventilating the inside of a building, likely to have its air used by many persons, has yet been discovered, which does not recognise the necessity for having large and direct openings to the outside air. The House of Commons, and some quite modernly-built Law Courts, University Examination Halls and Council Rooms, Theatres, and even Hospitals have no means whatever of getting fresh air directly into their interiors. They seem to be constructed on the erroneous assumption that the outside air is less fit to breathe than that

P. S.   5 which of necessity resides within a building. The greater the number in all classes of society who have been trained at sanatoriums in hygiene and the common sense of healthy living, the more quickly will woeful ignorance and gloomy prejudice in such matters be dispelled. The more quickly, too, will an outburst of political energy arise to insist on better housing conditions. The housing question cannot be settled by the efforts of a few enlightened reformers, or of keen County Councils and Medical Officers of Health here and there. The subject involves considerations connected with land values, rating, wages, imperial taxation, sanitation, means of transit, etc. Until the community at large appreciate better the various influences at work militating against better housing, and the means to bring about extensive alterations, little that is widely effective can be accomplished, in spite of present legislative powers.

(B) *The presence of the tubercle bacillus.* The influence of sanatoriums on the prevention of, and spread of, the tubercle bacillus is great. It is not the man who comes from a well-conducted sanatorium who is generally to be feared as a source of infection. He not only knows and practises the necessary precautions, but he also enlightens others. On the other hand, the untrained man in bad surroundings, often suffering from consumption which is undiagnosed, without knowledge of the evils of his surroundings or desire for their betterment, may be disseminating the disease broadcast.

It is surprising to find sometimes how inefficiently some patients deal with their expectoration when they have been under home treatment, even though they have had the benefit of medical advice from several sources, and how inadequately they learn the simple hygienic precautions necessary to observe, when tubercle bacilli are present in the sputum, in order to avoid infecting those in close contact with them. In this connection elementary instruction is also quite necessary to overcome the fears, often extreme and largely ill-founded, of infection. Sometimes people fear entering a sanatorium because they believe they become branded. They are afraid of social ostracism or loss of employment. Too often do ex-sanatorium patients who have recovered meet with such hardships, because there is generally no excuse for such treatment. Again the placing of a sanatorium in a neighbourhood is now-a-days usually strongly resented on the grounds that its presence is a danger to the public health of the district. Yet there are no good grounds for this fear. The Astor Departmental Committee in its final report (p. 4) well says, "a properly conducted institution is not a source of danger to the neighbourhood." Again, groundless misgivings are prevalent in some quarters when those who are merely suspected of having tuberculosis are recommended to take up their residence in a sanatorium amongst many persons known to have the disease. In reality the most suitable place for such people until they become quite well is in a sanatorium. Practically all suspects already have the germs of tuberculosis in them, and it is these they should fear. And a well-conducted sanatorium is, of all places, the safest; for there alone is it certain that all the simple precautions are taken, and there also fresh air and sunshine abound.

(C) *The present lack of means to ensure early diagnosis and adequate treatment.* Sanatorium treatment shows in a better way than anything else the essential dependence of medicine upon common-sense and upon the simple laws of hygiene. Constant reliance on common-sense and simple hygiene puts and keeps in their proper places intricate means of diagnosis, complicated methods of treatment, the use of drugs, and the amount of money and energy to expend on research. This influence of sanatoriums has always been conspicuous and is no less necessary now than of yore.

The knowledge of the methods by which the extinction of tuberculosis can be brought about is now such that steady and satisfactory advance towards the desired goal can be anticipated, so long as good use is made of present knowledge. That is, money and energy must be plentiful and well directed. Expenditure must not be too lavishly incurred in endeavours to find some new short-cut. The indebtedness of mankind to scientific research is great ; and pressing is the need for pursuing further investigations. But some seem to think no advance can be made except along the line of future research : this is a mistake. Also, if patients are treated at home science loses much of the valuable observation possible to collect in an institution. Therefore scientific investigations into the problems connected with tuberculosis which are still unsolved, can be pursued with more economy and efficiency if recourse is had to sanatorium treatment.

The influence of sanatorium treatment upon bringing about better means of ensuring an early diagnosis,
and the adequate treatment of tuberculosis, can best
be considered under the two divisions : (*a*) the education of the public, and (*b*) the education of the medical
profession.   Often now-a-days it is the ex-sanatorium
patient who helps others, sometimes, I regret to think,
more than the practitioner, to realise the importance of
early symptoms, of an examination of expectoration,
and of complete rest when slight fever is present.   But
default in this particular on the part of the doctor is frequently due more to misfortune than to fault.   Much
spade work has to be done in getting over all kinds of
prejudices amongst the people, in overcoming the
fanciful conceptions of tradition, and the touching faith
in medicines, especially when lauded in the advertisement columns of newspapers.   Even the distrust of
institutional treatment has to be coped with amongst
certain ignorant members of the working classes.   Sanatoriums are doing much to surmount these difficulties.

The present serious shortcomings of medical training
and experience in respect of sound and full knowledge
about tuberculosis have recently been repeatedly pointed
out, notably in the final report of the Astor Departmental Committee.   These shortcomings can be made
good by carrying out several reforms.   In the first
place more financial assistance from communal funds
must undoubtedly soon be forthcoming towards the
support of medical education in general, and towards
the expenses in particular of post-graduate study in
tuberculosis.   It is quite worth while to give money
to practitioners for the purpose of letting them gain

a short training in a sanatorium, as is done in parts of Norway. In the second place in the training of medical students certain reforms are palpably necessary. These have relation to : (*a*) the teaching, and (*b*) the teacher. Under the former head, more emphasis should be laid upon common diseases, upon the insepar-ability of prevention and cure, upon the importance of common-sense, and of the broad rules of hygiene. Under the latter head difficulties at once arise, for present arrangements in the United Kingdom, although seemingly stereotyped, may soon have to be altered ; yet they cannot be altered without a considerable revolution in the medical world.

I will but lay down a few propositions which seem to me to indicate to some extent the probable trend of events. The decline of medical charities seems likely to be progressive ; this being the case, the partnership of medical education with them will have to be modified or abandoned. Let it be noted, too, that it is particularly where medical teaching has often, up to the present, been deficient, that the separation be-tween medical charity and medical education is already becoming most immediate and complete. Especially is this noticeable in connection with tuberculosis. The consultant teacher of the present day combines the duties of visiting hospital patients and teaching in the hospital medical school, with the calling of con-sultant adviser, usually through general practitioners, to the well-to-do. From the nature of his duties and calling he is apt to be better as a diagnostician than as a preventer and curer of disease, and apt to place undue emphasis upon the purely technical side of medicine. So although many fine, practical teachers have been produced under this system, deficiencies in the capabilities of the teachers are apt to occur just where defects are most deplorable.

(D) *Social and industrial conditions affecting the food and work of the individual.* Phthisis is about two-and-a-half times more prevalent in the industrial than it is in the middle and upper classes. This fact is due more to the prevalence of unhealthy trades and low wages than to the greater opportunities for infection amongst the poorer classes. When people learn, partly through the influence of sanatoriums, that the trials of preventable disease can be added to the other hardships which they often compulsorily and silently endure as a result of poor wages, long hours, deficient food and housing, the demand for better social conditions will become more urgent. In many of these respects, the middle classes too have much to learn. For example, how late some persons are in learning that the human machine must have periodical and adequate leisure and rest. Some members of the professions and some independent traders have more to learn in this respect than many an artisan. Some people, especially women perhaps, seem never willing to put themselves "off duty," even when they are in a position to do so periodically and properly. A week or two in a good sanatorium generally teaches much in this respect.

CHAPTER IX

IN the future consumption will be extinct, and that will have been brought about largely through the efforts and influence of the chief factor, viz. the sanatorium, in the campaign against it. Meanwhile the gradually increasing regard for the worth of sanatoriums will lead to the treatment of patients suffering from other diseases than tuberculosis in institutions situated in clean country air, and governed by resident medical experts. This method will be extended, first to those suffering from other chronic or subacute maladies, and later to most of those suffering from acute illness, or accident. Even now in other lands some of those patients who are taken suddenly and acutely ill are removed, with marked advantage, from the centres of population to country hospitals: *e.g.* in New York infants seized with diarrhœa. When consumption has become extinct, therefore, sanatorium buildings may still be found useful. Future hospitals will probably be managed partly by the central government or municipality, partly by insurance societies, or authorities, and partly by an organised medical profession. A National Medical Service is not agreeable either to the doctors or to the people of this land. Compromise commends itself to English traditions. Changes must be gradual, and compromises may often be necessary. Whatever arrangements are made, the organic relationship and co-ordination of all medical services is essential, and medical treatment must be directly under the control of doctors alone. There can be no water-tight compartments; but this is not inconsistent with special institutions such as fever hospitals, asylums, sanatoriums, etc. In several countries on the continent there is already more movement towards the multiplication of special institutions than can be discerned at home.

Some of the most difficult reforms to inaugurate and complete will be in connection with medical education. The teaching capabilities of the best resident experts must be developed and used; and with this it will be well to associate arrangements by which the well-to-do can obtain the advantages of consultation with these doctors experienced in their special branches.

Sir R. W. Philip has said, " I would fain see parents insisting on the periodic examination of their children at home, and the periodic inspection of home conditions." It will devolve upon the general practitioner of the future to bring about this desirable end, and to apply the same principles to the whole population. Then doctors will become more completely divided into those who will be practitioners helping to prevent and diagnose disease, and those treating the sick in institutions for special diseases. But both divisions must be teachers of hygiene to a greater extent than is usually the case at the present time.

Increased knowledge shows more and more every day that the eradication of disease is a social problem. All parties in a modern state are animated by the serious aims, or show attachment to the cause, of social reform. Yet social legislation becomes a danger to the party which brings it in when weak and arbitrary administration, bringing disappointment and stirring up resentment, robs reforms of much of their efficiency and attraction. Meanness, the hostility of party political bias, and the creation by law of new vested interests, can do much to deprive sound social reform of its benefits, and to injure the party bringing it in. Let every citizen, actuated only by desire for the common good, bear his part, and show zeal and competence in the administration of reforms in order to gain the full advantages of them. The zealous are sometimes incompetent, and the competent not zealous. But careful study of social problems will bring much of both zeal and competence. With an appeal to the medical profession to be leaders in this study I lay down my pen.

APPENDIX I

Bibliography

My indebtedness to past writers is great, and it has been impossible to acknowledge it at all adequately in the text of my thesis. I have been influenced by study of the following books :

Bardswell, N. D. "The Consumptive Working Man."
—— "Advice to Consumptives."
—— "Diets in Tuberculosis."
—— "The Expectation of Life of the Consumptive after Sanatorium Treatment."
Brown, E. Vipont. "The Medical Profession."
Burton-Fanning, F. W. "The Open-air treatment."
Dodd, F. Lawson. "A National Medical Service."
Garland, C. H. "Insurance against Consumption."
Garland, C. H. and Lister, T. D. "Sanatoria for the People."
Gibbon, I. G. "Medical Benefit in Germany and Denmark."
Hutchinson, Woods. "Conquering Consumption."
Latham, A. and Garland, C. H. "The Conquest of Consumption."
Latham, A. "Prize Essay on the Erection of a Sanatorium."
Macdonald, J. R. "The Socialist Movement."
Mackenzie, W. Leslie. "Health and Disease."
McCormac, Hy. "On Pulmonary Consumption," 1855.
Moore, B. "The Dawn of the Health Age."
Newman, Sir G. "The Health of the State."
Newsholme, A. "The Prevention of Consumption."
Paterson, Marcus. "Auto-inoculation in Pulmonary Tuberculosis."
Walters, F. R. "Sanatorium treatment."
Webb, S. and B. "The State and the Doctor."
Woodcock, H. de C. "The Doctor and the People."

Besides the aid I have got from the study of the above books, I have been helped by government publications, and by innumerable articles and letters to the periodical press, medical and lay, and reference to even the more important of these is not possible.

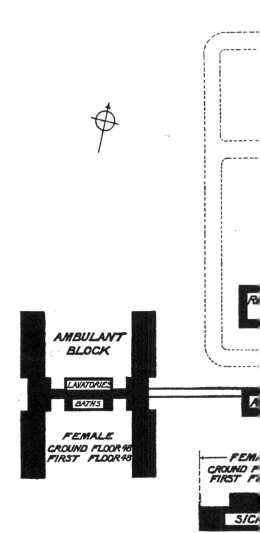

– *Sanatorium for 250 Patients* –
– *Block Plan* –

AMBULANT BLOCK

LAVATORIES

BATHS

FEMALE
CROUND FLOOR 48
FIRST FLOOR 48

FEM
CROUND F
FIRST F

SIC

SCALE OF

Plan I

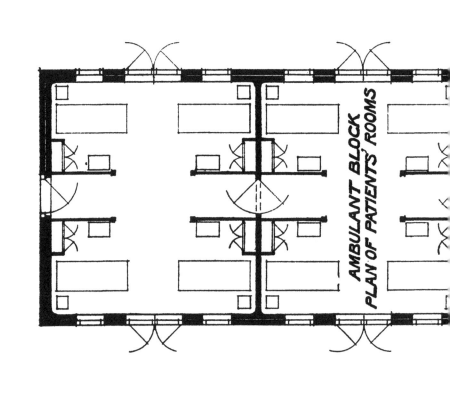

AMBULANT BLOCK
PLAN OF PATIENTS' ROOMS

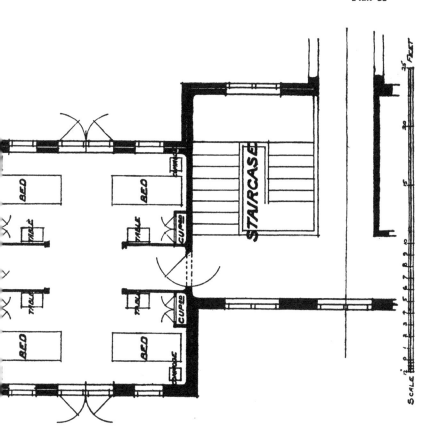

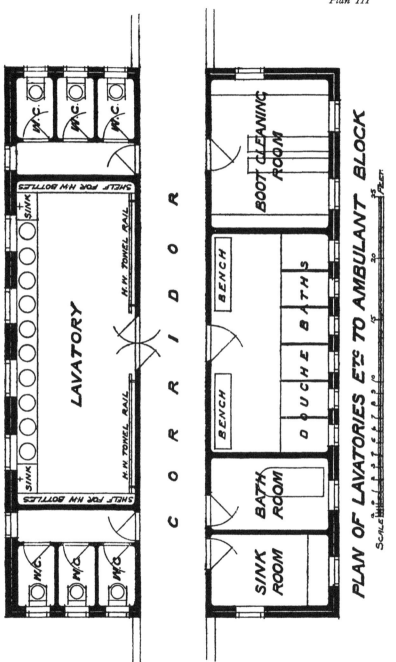

PLAN OF LAVATORIES ETC TO AMBULANT BLOCK

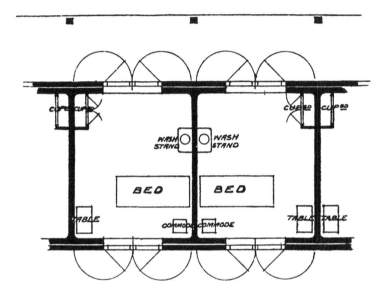

SICK BLOCK
PLAN OF PATIENTS ROOMS

SCALE ⊢⊢⊢⊢⊢⊢⊢⊢⊢⊢⊢ FEET.

INDEX